On Being Born

*Celebrating Life
Mothers and Medical Progress*

M J Badenhorst

First published in 2022 by
M.J. Badenhorst

M J Badenhorst
Wilmslow
Cheshire
United Kingdom
marthinus@btinternet..com

Being born is a good start

Table of contents

PROLOGUE..V

INTRODUCTION 7

A STUTTERED START..9

DANGEROUS PRESENCE 12

BORROWED BREASTS 15

VALUABLE ASSETS 18

A SHEER PLEASURE..21

I AM UNIQUE. WOW! 24

PROUD PLACENTALS 27

WHY WAS I WELCOMED? 31

A DELICATE BALANCE 34

WAS SHE SICK? 37

PAINFULLY PERPLEXED 40

WHAT WAS SHE THINKING 43

FEELING IT 46

NOT FEELING IT...49

PRAISE FOR THE POPPY AND THE COCA!..........................53

RELAX, IT'S NATURAL!..55

BREAKING THE SILENCE...58

PICTURE IMPERFECT..61

WOMB WITH A VIEW...64

A CUT BELOW...66

FORCEPSED OUT 69

SCISSORS, PLEASE! 72

A MATURE BABY? 76

IN SEARCH OF MY I 79

WELL CONNECTED 82

SOURCES AND FURTHER READING......................................85

Prologue

All people who have ever lived, from the nameless millions who lived in the dim and distant past to people whose names and faces are instantly recognisable by almost all of the more than seven billion of us living today, have one thing in common. They were all born from, and borne by a mother. Lift their shirts and the evidence is clear: they all have a belly button, an indisputable piece of evidence that they all once were attached to a woman via a tube. Cyrus, Caesar, Cleopatra, Christ, Mary, Mohammed, Marie Curie and Nelson Mandela along with everyone else who ever lived, was once conceived, was a fertilised egg, a very small diploid zygote of two cells, a morula of more cells, a blastocyst, a ball of cells which grafted itself onto the wall of a woman's womb. All of them, all of us, were embryos, grew into foetuses, lived in an amniotic sac for about two hundred and eighty days and eventually came down and out from between the legs of a woman whether it occurred in a primitive cave or in a comfortable place two million years or two minutes ago. Our one indisputable point of commonality is our natality. Nationality, a relatively recent development, defines our difference but our natality—natural, uninvented—defines our sameness.

All people, even the most feared, revered and most powerful who ever lived, dictators and despots, commanders, composers cooks and crazy people were once clueless, utterly helpless and totally dependent. They could not eat, they could not sit, they could not say anything. They could only speak the international lingua franca of all babies: crying, screaming, complaining and cooing. The best and the brightest who ever lived, Bach, Beethoven, the Beetles, Brian Cox and Maria Callas, all had to be potty trained prior to which they had no control over their bowels and bladder and no notion of a problem in that regard.

This book takes time to stop and think about the beginning no one can forget or remember.

Introduction

In the weeks after my dear mother's death, and probably as part of the grieving process, I devoted some time to think about her role in giving me the gift of life and what giving birth and being born actually entailed. I decided to discipline and organise my thinking by producing short essays about various related subjects and this book is the result. I started with my own story, broadening out to interesting aspects of the history and science involved. I am not medically trained, my background is in theology, but I tried nonetheless to think and write clearly to make it edifying as well as entertaining to anyone who has ever been born or who has given birth, or maybe going to sometime in the future. That's a big potential audience! Of course, anyone who wants to know more will do well to consult the professionals and their writings. The chapters can all be read as stand-alone pieces.

Mum and I didn't get off to a great start (A Stuttered Start). The doctor did not show up and this was very traumatic to my mother. Then her (my!) milk was late and I was fortunately fed by 'Borrowed Breasts' for which I should of course be very grateful. This story set me thinking about the value of these 'Valuable Assets' after which the whole family of mammals are named. The story of the absent doctor as 'A Dangerous Presence' when doctors were the cause of death in many instances until the science developed to understand what was going on. 'Sheer Pleasure' is about the marvellous thought that I was the result of two people making love. Looking at DNA and ordinary finger printing techniques, I was astonished to discover that no two people are fully identical, not even identical twins. It is a mind-blowing thought: I am Unique, Wow! In 'Proud Placentals' I discover this valuable organ, so special, that some people think we could easily have been called placentals instead of mammals. The next two chapters look at survival of the unborn. 'Why was I welcomed, 'is about the amazing exception the immune system makes for the new, and half foreign growth which would otherwise be attacked and eliminated. Sometimes pregnancy needs to be terminated for medical reasons. But this of course leads into the big debate about abortion. I don't go into it deeply, just touch on it and suggest a Delicate Balance needs to be struck. I think with compassion about the difficulty and the pain my mother endured giving birth to me and it led me to ask why childbirth is so difficult. For most other mammals it appears to be much easier and mostly far less dangerous. Three chapters are devoted to aspects surrounding why birth is so painful before turning attention to ways of mitigating pain and making delivery easier including C-section and other surgical procedures that help to make things easier. I was gobsmacked to learn that in our desire to be able to see the condition of the unborn, mother's and foetuses were routinely subjected to X-Ray imaging with disastrous consequences. Fortunately, Ultra-Sound technology came along and saved the day and many lives. I was a mature, that is full term baby, but my one grandson was born eleven weeks prematurely. Sometimes foetuses don't perform the natural turning dance to be born and these breech births are delicate matters that need to be handled with care and skill. Finally in the twenty-fifth chapter I look away from my/our uniqueness to our astonishing connectedness with just about everyone and everything else.

As I remember my mother, I also hail Mother Nature and all our marvellous mothers.

1

A Stuttered Start

My birth was a bit of a mess. They never are particularly easy, neat and tidy experiences. No experience that involves bleeding and pain can ever be elegant and pleasant. Although I was there and very much involved, I have no recollection of it of course. I do have memories though, based on the first-hand experience of someone who was there through it all, my mother. This was a time when I really needed her. I am really glad she was there. Of course, it wasn't optional. I am no expert, but I think there has never been a birth where the mother was absent. Unconscious, dead even, but not physically absent. My mother was physically present and conscious throughout the whole event. She remembered certain aspects vividly. Not pleasant, and really scary for mother and baby.

The scariest thing of several scary things was that the doctor didn't show up. He wasn't there. He promised he'd be there, but when the moment came, he wasn't. Apparently, he had calculated that the birth was still a while away, enough time for him to quickly perform an operation on some other patient, I think it may well have been tonsils or appendix. This was the heyday of tonsillectomies, almost every child who ever got a sore throat or more than two colds per season, was a prime candidate for the top treatment for all these conditions: a tonsillectomy. And for some reason every second person with a stomach-ache anywhere approaching the right side of the body, was equally a prime candidate for an appendectomy. From a business perspective, bearing in mind that doctors were almost all in private practice which meant they had a business to run and a profit to turn, these quick and easy solution surgeries were good sources of income. I am not saying that all the people who underwent these procedures didn't need them, or that they didn't benefit from them, but it is rather interesting to note that today these procedures are rarely performed. Anyway, someone, the doctor, the patient or both needed one of these while my mother and I were in labour. The two of us wanted the same thing. I wanted to be out, and she also wanted me out. You could say I wanted to be outed as a human being! I was fed up being a foetus and frankly was beginning to be a right pain in a place for my mother.

There was no one else, at least no one experienced and equipped to deal with a birth. There was only a very inexperienced trainee nurse in her first month who advised my mother to keep the whole thing to herself. 'Don't push! 'She pleaded. Not a great combination: the end of the last month of a pregnancy and the beginning of a first month of general nursing training! She had no clue what to do and apparently told everybody about it, loud and clear. Petrified and panicky she promenaded up and down the corridors claiming impotence through ignorance. The place seemed to be deserted. There was no one knowledgeable to be found. And even my father wasn't there. Those were the days when dads were not allowed at births. They had to leave it all in the hands of the able albeit sometimes absent doctors and in the un-able and untrained hands of student nurses.

We did it by ourselves, mum and I, mostly mum, I think. And there I lay, shivering, whimpering and turning blue, with no blanket over me in a cold, country hospital in mid-October, still attached to my mother via the umbilical cord. I get shivers down my mature spine just thinking about it, but what a harrowing experience it must have been for her! The memories etched into her mind that day I never acquired. I am glad we both survived this stuttered start for me to tell the story.

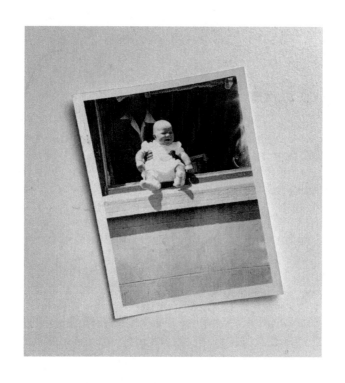

Here I am smiling at nobody in particular
at the age of 3 months and three weeks.

2

Dangerous Presence

My mother struggled to forgive the doctor who was absent at the crucial moment of delivery when she needed him. She never forgot and she told me the tale several times during her life. But there was a time when present doctors were more dangerous than absent ones. And there was also a long time when doctors weren't welcome to attend and even prohibited from attending births. There is a story about a certain doctor Wert who slipped into a delivery room in 1522 disguised as a woman. Apparently, he was a better doctor than a disguise artist because his cover was blown and he was kicked out by the disgusted women. The story even continues that he was prosecuted and killed. So attending was dangerous for the doctor!

In 1847 a Hungarian doctor by the name of Ignaz Semmelweis was working in Vienna where he noticed a very high rate of deaths due to so-called puerperal fever, childbed fever. He noticed that doctors and students were moving from autopsies to deliveries and came up with the idea that there had to be some connection. This was a time when germ theory of disease was still being developed. He thought it had something to do with cadavers, that somehow death was contagious and that the doctors were bringing it from the mortuary to the delivery room. His colleagues didn't take kindly to the suggestion they might be the problem. They took it very personally. How in the world could they, the healers, be the killers! What outrageous and offensive nonsense! Paradigms don't shift easily.

So, Dr. Semmelweis conducted an experiment. He instructed all doctors and students who came from autopsies to wash their hands in a chlorinated liquid and to his relief the death rate dropped from 20 to 2%, which must have been a tremendous relief to the women. And so, Dr. Semmelweis was honoured with something like a Nobel Prize for his breakthrough discovery, the discovery that doctors once literally had death on their hands. No, not at all, quite the opposite, he was criticised very harshly and attacked, and he landed in a mental asylum where he was also assaulted and died. He got it wrong. Death wasn't contagious. It wasn't the fault of the deceased. But he also had it quite right that it was something deadly on the hands of the doctors and that the healers were the killers, serial killers in fact.

It is quite amazing that these doctors gave Dr. Semmelweis such a hard time in 1847, because two hundred years before around 1640, the Dutchman Antonie van Leeuwenhoek, today generally regarded as one of the fathers of microbiology, had already seen little 'animals' under the lens of his microscope. It seems that the penny was slow to drop for these doctors. It was only when the real heavyweights, the trilogy of Louis Pasteur, Robert Koch and Joseph Lister (among others) weighed in with their careful research that the reality of this unseen world of powerful pathogens became clear. Today sterilisation is routine and although infections still occur, the risks are far better understood and prevented.

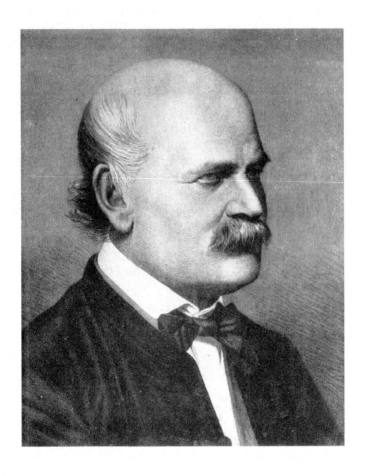

Dr. Ignaz Semmelweis - 1 July 1818 - 13 August 1865

Maybe mother and I were better off without the doctor there that day.

3

Borrowed Breasts

In the hours and days following my birth a new threat appeared. A food shortage! No, there wasn't a famine of biblical proportions in the little Highveld, country town of Amersfoort in South Africa. It wasn't a case of the hospital running low on supplies. No, the white gabled Elsie Ballot hospital had enough food for all of its patients. Some didn't need much because after a tonsillectomy you can only eat jelly and ice cream. It was infant me. There wasn't enough food for me, a problem about which the hospital's kitchen couldn't do anything. I couldn't even eat some of the tonsillectomy jelly. I couldn't eat anything, really. I needed milk, a mother's milk. I had a mother, she survived the birth, but her milk had not arrived yet. I am not sure how these things work, whether someone needs to fill in a form and pre-order and whether the bureaucratic business was botched, I don't know. I simply wasn't abreast with all of this and neither was mother, quite literally. I wasn't happy. And of course, as you can imagine, my mum was also rather frustrated with her own milk production. She really wanted to feed me.

Fortunately, a day or so after my birth another woman gave birth to her baby and apparently, she had ample supply. She had enough for twins but as she didn't have twins I was twinned with her baby. If you think that twinning towns from different countries is nonsense and that it doesn't really work, this form of twinning worked a treat. My mum says she was a bit envious of this woman's productive prowess and my dad was also rather impressed. Mother had ambivalent feelings about it, very grateful on the one hand, and rather sad too, because there I was on the other woman's breast having the time of my life. She felt a bit cheated. She couldn't blame me, of course, I wasn't cheating, I was just eating.

I never knew the name of this bountiful benefactor who saved my life with her breasts. Mother never mentioned her name, or any other details. Just unhelpful little things like the fact that she had black, curly hair and that one breast was bigger than her baby's head. I am not sure how relevant that is. By not knowing who she was, I could never thank her or be embarrassed by anyone bringing this fact up in conversation, but I do feel a debt of gratitude to this anonymous woman. I was just one, but to me it was as important as the feeding of the five thousand, maybe more important.

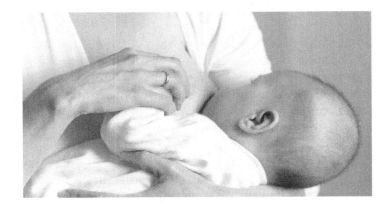

[*Image:* Freepik.com]

So, I honestly want to pay homage to a fellow human who single handedly broke a famine for me and fed me with the most important meals of my life. People have given me meals during my life, fillet steak and baked potato, my granny's sourdough bread with butter and jam, a stack of pancakes on a rainy day, a quick burger and chips in later years when American fast food invaded our culture, hearty, traditional Christmas dinners, so many delicious and often indulgent meals, but none of them was as welcome and as beneficial as mother's milk from an unknown woman in the first week of my life.

4

Valuable Assets

I am truly grateful to the woman who's breasts were borrowed to feed me when my mother's milk production was delayed, and to this day, I confess, breasts are beautiful to me. But it is not only me. Breasts are beautiful to most men, a fact which has not gone unnoticed and unappreciated by women. A culture with a long history has developed around putting them on display. Evening dresses are designed with them in mind and women wear them proudly and provocatively at glamorous events like film festivals and formal dinners. Breasts are still used to sell things. One might even succumb to the temptation of calling this use of it, booby traps! When, in the eponymous film Erin Brockovich (played by Julia Roberts) she manages to obtain valuable, obscure information and her incredulous boss asks how she managed to do it, she responds, 'they're called boobs, Ed!' Until very recently a tabloid newspaper in the UK reserved its page three for them and of course all their male readers who eagerly turned to page three first. To us as mammals breasts are good news and men can't get enough of them. Our culture, in spite of all of the recent developments regarding depiction of women are still a bit obsessed with breasts. And we are not the only ones!

Turn the pages of history and you will see the same thing. Breasts on display, on canvasses, in sculptures and photographs. And it is not just hedonistic cultures, but very religious ones too. Goddesses like Astarte with prominent breasts were publicly displayed and worshiped. Isis, the Egyptian goddess is often depicted as the benevolent one who fed future Pharaohs at her breast. Greek culture loved the body in its nude form in general and although many of the gods were boys, they had some lovely girls too, Gaia, Hera and Artemis and of course, don't forget Aphrodite-Venus, the goddess of love, always portrayed fully nude. And think of the image of the virgin and the baby Jesus and his mother. Some of the most intimate images are of the little Lord sucking at the breast of the Mother of God.

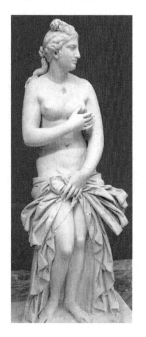

But our involvement with breasts is much older and more basic than this. Don't forget that we are mammals, which refers to the mammary gland, that is, the breast. We (mammals) evolved about 300 million years ago and we have two important characteristics, live birth and breastfeeding. No wonder that the most intimate name for the one with the mammaries is simply, mamma. Our big brain development as primates and later as sapiens came a lot later, which means that breasts precede our brains by millions of years! No wonder we find them erogenous.

The development of breasts in the individual human is a clear sign that the female is ready to be a mother and of course males get the message that they might be ready to mate. Some psychologists have thought that the size of the breasts spell fertility in the brain of the male, but more recent studies have indicated that it might be more basic than that. Men find them alluring no matter the size and even the shape. This attention and attraction are probably the driving force behind women going to great lengths and expense to elect for cosmetic surgery, boob jobs, as they are called colloquially.

The problem however is not physical enhancement or reduction, but rather the social and psychological reduction, the attitude whereby women are reduced to baby making bodies with boobs. Society is discovering to its great benefit

19

that women can be as brainy as any man and still breastfeed a baby. We need to get the balance right on brains and breasts.

Both are valuable assets.

5

A Sheer Pleasure

My father was absent during my birth but he was present when it counted. At my conception. I am grateful for that. My birth was a pain, but my conception was a pleasure. I am the product of love. I am my parents' love child. I have evidence for this. I have seen the photographs of them clearly in love, like the one below. I have read some of the letters my father wrote. I didn't know he had it in him to wax so romantic. I don't need much evidence though; I am the evidence, and it is nice to know my parents found pleasure in producing me.

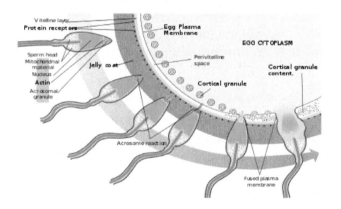

[Image: [LadyofHat, Wikipedia]

It is a precious thing to ponder without being impolite to my parents. An hour or so before I was conceived there was lovely love making with the juices flowing resulting in a sudden release of sperm, little tadpole-like things, about two hundred and fifty million of them each programmed with a single purpose in mind, not that they have much of a mind, to get to the egg. They are equipped with something a little bit like a GPS, a little sat-nav to guide them. The conditions themselves are not easy to navigate.

It is not like little fish swimming in water, it is more like jelly and there are waves and currents.Imagine surfing on a sea of jelly, a turbulent sea of jelly. Hit the wave, or rather be hit by the wave, at the wrong moment and get sloshed sideways out of the mainstream, or worse backwards causing loss of valuable time, and it is a race! Hit the wave just right however and get projected forward improving chances in the race. Sperm are not good swimmers. They don't really swim properly like competent fish. At best they zig-zag. They do their best though, but they are slow. On their own, at top speed, they can manage about 3 millimeters per minute. Fortunately, the tide and the movements inside help to pull some of them in. Nevertheless, of the quarter of a billion that set off only about 10% get close to the target. The fatality rate is phenomenal. Once the few exhausted survivors reach the target another difficult obstacle awaits, getting through the tough wall of the egg. Out of 250 million hopefuls one, just one, makes it in and once it is in, the wall hardens to quash the hopes of any other triers. Game over! But it is only the end of the beginning signalling the start of a new, unique individual. This primordial odyssey took place while my two loving parents were sleeping. It was a pleasure making me, I am sure.

My lovely, loving parents before they got married

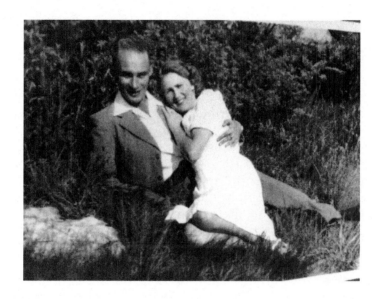

6

I am Unique. Wow!

It is an astounding thought that I am unique. Out of more than seven billion people it is possible to identify me because I am different from all of them. I even stand out uniquely from every Homo Sapiens who ever walked this planet! In the fertilised egg that developed into me 23 chromosomes came from the single sperm cell that my father contributed, bequeathed to me. The Y on the last chromosome, chromosome 23 came from him which made me male. The other 23 chromosomes came from my mother. In the genes on the long ladder of DNA in my father's chromosomes are not only contained all the information to build a human body, but it also contains all the little idiosyncrasies of my father's family line. And the same applies to the copies of genes I received from my mother. I inherited family traits from her family as well. There are things about me and my body that are determined by heredity from each of these familial lines. My father, although intimately associated with my mother and therefore her history, does not possess a family relationship with my mother or her family. And again, the same applies to my mother and how she relates to my father and his family. They relate socially, maybe psychologically and culturally, even biologically because they are both human of course, but in terms of the genetic differences associated with heredity, they are not related. But I am. That makes me more related to my father and mother than they are to each other. In spite of this relatedness and intimacy the package I have inherited is unique.

This fact is powerfully underscored by Dactyloscopy, the fancy word for fingerprinting and the genetic equivalent of DNA 'fingerprinting' or profiling both of which are routinely used in forensic research. Fingerprints are tiny friction ridges and valleys at the end of each finger formed during a baby's time in the womb. There is a one in 64 billion chance of two individuals having identical fingerprints. Not even identical twins have the same fingerprints.

The pattern of lines on the skin of my fingers were formed around the tenth to seventeenth week of pregnancy when I, inside of my mother, was about four to eight centimeters long, about the size of my thumb. The basal layer bends and buckles, forming loops, whorls and arches or ridges and these touch-patterns are as permanent as they are unique because no two foetuses, 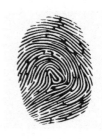 not even identical twins, have the same touch history. These patterns are there for life and is reproduced reliably when the outward layers of skin is damaged. Just think of this for a second, I could be positively identified as having been on a crime scene when I was a boy as big as my thumb! I plead innocent, however.

DNA profiling developed over recent decades provides an even stronger source of uniqueness. It is based on the sequencing and analysis of minute variables in the gene code. It is a complicated process and there are different methods of doing it, but it is now so refined and mechanised that it can produce a result in a matter of minutes. Our genome is 99.9% identical, but there are many, small idiosyncrasies and it is possible, based on these minute variations to tell with a very high degree of probability that it belongs to a specific and unique individual.

On top of the biological and genetic data, the nature aspect, comes the nurture, the environmental, societal aspect, the way I as a unique individual relate to my unique surroundings and are shaped and formed by them. My environment, my nurture, is vastly different from that of my father and mother a generation before, even from my brother or other siblings. Even twins who grow up in the same environment have distinct aspects of their environmental interaction that are different. They don't get exactly the same academic scores, they don't display the same talents or inclinations and as a result the interactions are different, almost as different as the fingerprint patterns and the variations in the gene code.

I am just bowled over again, as I write this, to think that of all the people who have ever lived and all the people living today, billions of them, I am unique. I am special, not because I think so or believe it to be so, but because it is a simple, scientifically established fact. Wow!

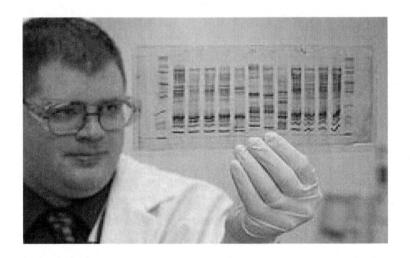

7

Proud Placentals

A few minutes after my birth the third stage of the birth process occurred, the expulsion of the placenta. I am not sure how it went, but in final analysis it must have been fine. No one is particularly impressed with the placenta. It is the afterbirth and an afterthought. No one turns from the newborn and the mother to think about the placenta. 'Here's the baby, and the tired but happy mum and here's a nice picture of the placenta!' The placenta is not photogenic. It is really ugly. It is a bloody mess. At least in its expelled afterbirth form.

It must have looked liked a kind of flat cake, because that's what the word placenta means. It comes from the Greek word meaning flat and the idea migrated into the Latin term *placenta uterine.* It means flat cake of the uterus, but it is absolutely nothing like a cake of any kind.

If we pause to ponder the placenta even for a little bit we discover the very valuable, vital functions this ugly organ performs at the most crucial time of our personal history and we also discover a fascinating piece of our evolutionary history. Before placentas there were eggs, as there still are. Most animals are oviparous, reproducing by means of fertilised eggs. This includes birds, reptiles and many other species. The egg is a little care package, a ration pack for the developmental journey. Apart from the delivered package nothing more comes from the mother. But we are so-called viviparous animals, growing the live baby inside of our bodies. We are mammals, but equally defining, we are placentals.

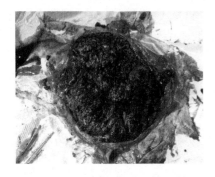

About a hundred and fifty million years ago a concestor[1] of ours, maybe a fury little fellow, managed to evade all of the dangerous, gigantic predators, but ironically got invaded by a minuscule, microbial agent, a virus looking for a host to trick into making copies of itself and to pass them on along the reproductive ride through time. And when microbiologists arrived at the ability of looking at our human genome in detail, they discovered amongst other things a strange, out of place RNA gene that looked like it belonged to a virus, a retrovirus group identified as ERVFRD-1. It encodes for a protein called syncytin-2. This protein is uniquely responsible for building the outer layer of the placenta, the border wall between foetus and mother. It has been given the tongue twister: syncytiotrophoblast. Try saying that before you have your first cup of coffee in the morning! It is really lucky for us this virus infected our ancient concestor because evolution used it to construct the placenta.

So, what did my placenta ever do for me? As the interface between two human individuals, the busy border crossing, it served to regulate, to import, to inspect and police and to provide. I needed oxygen but couldn't yet breathe because I was under water. The placenta enabled oxygen from my mother's breathing to get through to me without letting the blood streams get mixed. That would have been the end. I didn't have food and couldn't eat, but there again, the placenta by means of the umbilical cord let nutrients from my mother's diet pass through to me so I could grow and get ready for birth. Of course, carbon-dioxide and other waste products needed to be got rid of and again, the placenta did it. The placenta served to protect from attack, including from the mother's immune

---

[1] Richard Dawkins' term for a shared ancestor

system and it produces and provides several very helpful hormones, each doing very helpful things to protect and build the baby. It does it every moment of every day for around 280 days, 40 weeks, or nine months, day and night. And then, right at the end, as an afterbirth, having worked so well to get rid of waste products, it becomes one itself.

Usually and routinely in the West it lands in a dish destined for destruction with other human waste products. That's the way it goes, but not always and everywhere. Some cultures are different and treat the placenta with respect and almost reverence, and even in the West a new appreciation is growing leading to a variety of possible options. Some people take it home and consume it. That's right, cook and eat it! Or it is turned into tablets or powder and taken like supplements. It is also turned into a salve, a kind of cream. Some, following certain cultural traditions bury it with dignity, maybe with or next to a tree planted to mark the baby's birth. In some cases, it is even dried and formed into a picture frame for the baby. Yes, the placenta is kept in the picture after parturition (birth) by turning it into a picture frame. Interesting.

Placenta

I am not going to do any of these things, but I am doing my bit by praising the placenta for being such a wonderful shield and gatekeeper for me when it mattered most. And to think it became part of us through a viral infection and now here we are proud placentals!

Placenta en. wikipedia.org (accessed June 2020)

Mi, S., Lee, X., Li, X. *et al.* Syncytin is a captive retroviral envelope protein involved in human placental morphogenesis. *Nature* **403,** 785–789 (2000).

8

Why was I welcomed?

Around the time I was born in Africa a British scientist was wondering why I wasn't rejected. He wasn't thinking why my parents wanted me, or why my mother did not consider ending the pregnancy even if she could. And to be fair, he wasn't thinking of mother and me specifically, but mothers and embryos generally. He was contemplating what became known as the immunological paradox regarding pregnancy. He was thinking and researching a lot about immune response and seeing how our bodies possess the peculiar ability to identify 'own' and 'other' cells. Foreign cells trigger a fierce immune response. The body calls up an army of responders to attend the scene of the invasion, seal it off and put the invaders out of action. We have some really effective and deadly agents in our anatomical armoury who are engineered to kill, and they do not need a lot of provocation and persuasion. But why do embryos escape?

This paradox vexed Sir Peter Medawar. He had seen first-hand how our bodies reject a so-called allograft. An autograft, transplanting tissue from one part of the body to another part of the same body seems fine. Our bodies don't get inflamed and all worked up about it, but try this with tissue from another body and the proverbial breaks loose. Persuading the body's immune system to accept an allograft is quite an ask. So, why is the body okay with a blastocyst, a ball of cells, grafting itself, implanting

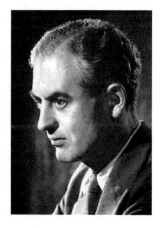

itself, into the lining of the uterus considering that half of its building material are from a different human being? Why does the mother's immune system acquiesce, making this an exceptional case?

When I was safely out of the womb and about ten years old Doctor Medawar was highly praised, even awarded the Nobel Prize along with Frank Burnet from Australia in 1960 for pioneering work in tissue grafting which is the basis of organ transplants, and for their discovery of acquired immunological tolerance.

Although his proposals and solutions to this problem did not stand the test of time in science, he did ask the right sort of question and it did rally the scholarly troops to work hard at the problem, knowing that if they could understand it, it could also go a long way towards making organ transplants work, which they realised could be a lifesaver in many desperate situations where organs failed or were damaged beyond repair.

The results of decades of research by many dedicated professionals is quite extensive and really technical. First and foremost, there is the syncytial security wall that operates in and from the placenta. It seems to create what has been called an 'immune privileged' site where perceived antigens are somehow tolerated without triggering the inflammatory response. Another important role creating an environment of tolerance is played by Regulatory T-cells, called Tregs. And then there is the role of NK cells, natural killer cells! Their role is rather similar to the cytotoxic T-cells. They do what it says in their job description. They eliminate enemies for a living. But the NK's that operate in the uterus, called uNK cells act uncharacteristically. They seem to have the uncanny ability to 'read' paternal antigens as 'our', 'not-other' and therefore they do not target the cells coming from the father.

The research results are very technical and complicated to the untrained and there is far more to this than (literally) meets the eye, but it seems clear that there is a quite complex set of factors, not just a single, simple one, all 'talking to each other' in order to make an exception to the rule of attacking paternal antigens and killing them. Metaphorically speaking the killer squads are not called up because a moratorium on aggression, a temporary truce is created chemically in order to allow the foetus to remain a welcomed, not vilified guest within its host's body. In a sense we function a bit like a virus and it is vital otherwise viviparity would not work. Fortunately, it does.

But not always. Sometimes this friendly, tolerant environment changes into the fierce area of conflict again. In the case of Rh disease, the mother produces antibodies against the Rhesus-D on her baby's red blood cells. It happens when the mother is Rh-negative, and the baby is Rh-positive. It is 'noticed' by the body in a first pregnancy and antibodies are made, but the placenta forms an effective barrier resulting in a normal pregnancy. But as soon as a second pregnancy occurs, the alarms go off and the security squads come rushing in, the mother's antibodies, this time able to cross the placental barrier and attack the very vulnerable foetus' red blood cells. Effective screening can provide prevention, treatment and a good outcome.

Another negative response against the placenta is called pre-eclampsia (PE). It is characterised by high blood pressure. It usually occurs at about the half-way point of pregnancy. If untreated it can be severe leading to seizures, multiple organ distress and failure and also the loss of the pregnancy, in this case called eclampsia.

Given how dangerous the early environment in the uterus could be and how aggressive and intolerant a human body can be to an allograft, I am very grateful for the creation of a clement climate by the intricate interactions of the two bodies.

I am really grateful I was welcomed, not rejected.

9

A Delicate Balance

When my mother became pregnant with me, it was her egg and my father's sperm which found each other and formed a union. It happened in her body. If she developed a different kind of growth, not a gestation, a tumour for instance, no one would deny 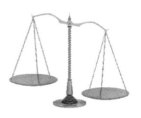 that she had the right, even the responsibility to have it removed, safely of course. But a tumour would never grow to be able to drive a train, pilot a plane or transplant a heart. Although it grows in her body, it is also a new body being grown there.

Societies that allow abortions have reached a compromise striking a delicate balance between the right of the baby and that of the mother. And the point of balance seems to be viability. Before that point a baby could not survive birth, but thereafter it is possible.

In England where I live that point is 23 weeks and 6 days. Up to this point medical practitioners are allowed to help a woman to terminate her pregnancy, but after it, they are not, and it becomes illegal. A woman can request an abortion at 23 weeks, but at 25 weeks she cannot. At that time society stands up for the unborn child against the woman, whereas society stood on the side of the mother and her rights up to that critical watershed.

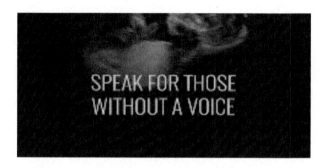

This is highly unsatisfactory to those who are adamant that life starts at conception and that no one has the right to terminate human life. These advocates want society to stand with the baby even before it is viable as a baby. To them viability is merely an arbitrary point that should not take precedence over the significant, even sacred moment of conception when (new) life starts. These advocates do not even exempt unwanted or violently enforced pregnancies as in the case of rape as reason to disregard the fact that wanted or not, life has started.

The other side of this controversy maintain that forcing women to go ahead with unplanned and unwanted pregnancies is unfair to women and potentially very bad for such an unwanted baby. They also contend that unprofessional 'back street' abortions could be very detrimental and dangerous, that abortions ought to be regulated and done professionally or not at all. They also point out that abortions are now quite safe and that it does not entail any suffering to mother or the foetus.

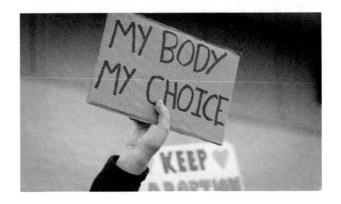

It is a difficult debate and a delicate balance to strike.

10

Was She Sick?

So there we were, mother and I. In the Elsie Ballot Hospital in Amersfoort. She, in a room in a bed with a really big, swollen-up belly and I, inside of her, the cause of the big bump on her belly. As the contractions intensified and became more frequent, the discomfort and pain increased. She was anxious and worried and in dire need of medical and nursing care, the absence of the doctor and the inexperience of the young nurse only contributing to the severity of her situation.

Why is that so, exactly? Was she sick? Was I making her sick at this early stage of our relationship? Did my father with all of that tender moments and loving attention cause her to contract something dangerous, some malady, the mother malady? Is it not a natural, simple and safe thing? One would think that procreating, adding some members to the family should be a fairly normal thing, not something to fear and fret about? We have been doing it, over and over again since time immemorial, for millions of years and we are the most evolved, most sophisticated, smartest species on the planet. Surely, we should have got better at it over time. Practice makes perfect. Why then was she in hospital where the sick people go and where the healers and nurses work? This is where people who had motor vehicle accidents go, people who suffered a stroke or a heart attack. I once saw a man in that same hospital who got caught in a runaway fire on his farm. He was badly burnt. These things are not normal. To get crushed in a car crash, to suffer a brain bleeding, blood flooding your head, or your heart stopping, or your skin burnt off your body, is not normal for human beings. They are catastrophes and of course you need to get to a hospital where doctors and nurses need to step in and see what can be done to these disruptions, these abnormalities. But is the lovely thing of having a baby in the same ballpark? Shouldn't having a baby be a normal and relatively easy thing? Who designed it to be so difficult and dangerous?

Roll back the reel of time and the Elsie Ballot doesn't exist. Roll back further and hospitals do not exist. Roll back some more and doctors are idiots, not having a clue and not worth the name doctor. And even further back, no doctors, at all, maybe a guy with some bones and stones. For at least two million years humans walked the planet, wandering after food and seeking shelter in caves, no houses, no shops, no specialists. The Einstein of prehistory was a guy who could make a pointy stone into a stone axe or tie a stone to a stick. And yet, they were having babies. Not the guy, his wife of course. They couldn't get angry at the doctor's absence, because all doctors were absent, always, because they didn't exist yet.

And if we look sideways to other animals, they don't have help at birth. The Giraffe or Zebra community doesn't seem to think the expecting mother Giraffe or Zebra are sick when the time comes to deliver their young. They just stand around chewing and before anyone can fuss the foal falls out. After a bit of licking and nibbling, the little fellow gets on his all fours, finds his mother's teat and starts to eat. No giraffe gynaecology required, zero help for the Zebra. Not a big deal. Looking left and right around us in nature we can observe with envy how those silly monkeys, baboons and apes get their babies, precariously perched high up in a tree. The mother does it all on her own and the infant is dextrous and strong and able to get swinging with mum and the rest of the troupe.

Why do we as humans and particularly modern humans have such precarious and painful births? Why did having me land her in hospital in desperate need of a doctor? Why didn't she just, you know, have me? Why did she get sick with me?

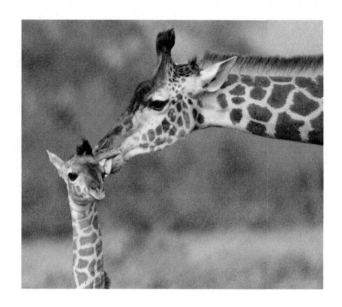

The Giraffe mother gives birth standing up. She pushes the calf out and the newborn falls about six feet, the fall breaking the umbilical cord. The mother cleans the calf and nudges it to stand up. After a few hours it is capable of running around.

11

Painfully Perplexed

People have been perplexed by the problem of pain during childbirth for a long time in our culture. For many centuries people looked to the Bible for answers and the Bible have always, well, delivered so to speak. You don't have to go very deep into the Good Book to find a specific answer to the problem of pain during childbirth. It is right there in chapter 3 of the very first book. God is angry with Eve, the first woman, because she disobeyed his rule. He puts a curse on Eve and all of her offspring, all women of the future.

"I will greatly multiply Your pain in childbirth, In pain you will bring forth children;
(New American Standard Bible)

'I will make your pains in childbearing very severe; with painful labor you will give birth to children.
(New International Version)
Genesis 3:16

There we have it. The origin is God: 'I will make your pains...very severe.' And there we also have the origin of the term 'labour' for giving birth, and the term 'labour pains.' The pain is punishment and the cause of it is sin. The woman brought it on herself and not only did she bring this pain upon herself and all of her female offspring, but she is also the cause of the curse on all humanity. Giving birth is painful, because it ought to be, because it is ordained to be. Every painful birth and every birth pain is a painful reminder of the rebellion of Eve and of the consequences of sin. Women should therefore carry this curse and its consequences without complaining contemplating the state of the human condition. Complaining, questioning or attempting to evade it, one runs the risk of a second disobedience. Over centuries these and similar sentiments have been drawn directly from this passage.

The influence of the Bible and passages like these has been substantial, built upon and perpetuated by influential church fathers, like Tertullian and Protestant reformers like Luther. But, surely, no one in their right mind can still find this explanation compelling and plausible today! Apparently, not so. A female theologian, in a recent article considers Luther's very influential views:

"Luther wants Christians to see the struggles of labor as something that God wills for a positive good, not as a negative sign. Birthing labor is actually a sign precisely of obedience to God's will...Facing the symptoms of the curse with courage and stamina, according to Luther, not only brings defeat of the devil. It also brings about God's promise to never abandon humanity...women are placed in a position to participate in God's creative processes in a way that only pregnant and birthing women can" (Amy Marga, Luther Seminary, St Paul, 2020)

A bible teacher on the Web accepts without question and promotes the literal interpretation of this bible text, saying:

"This judgement from God was meant to be one that every childbearing woman would experience. Pain in childbirth was placed on Eve and on every future mother. This pain serves as a universal reminder of God's judgment for the sin Adam and Eve brought into the world." (gotquestions.org)

And a young, modern Christian woman, Sarah Scherf writes in Christianity Today:

41

"But here's the thing: Natural childbirth is really, really excruciating. While I understand that many women indeed feel empowered by delivering new life into the world, I don't share the feeling. Childbirth is the most painful, breaking experience I have ever had. And, I must remember, why shouldn't it be?" Quoting Genesis 3:16 she concludes: *"Like my sister, Eve, I am under the Curse."* (Christianity Today Feb. 2014)

Really? Isn't this a case of adding insult to injury? Not only do women have to endure the excruciating physical pain associated with childbirth, but they also have to accept that it is a curse placed on them, that the curse is their fault, that they should therefore stoically accept it and even thank God because it is his will and part of his plan of salvation. That is a lot to stomach! All the more reason for bible readers to consider critically the genre of the literature involved as well as the historical context of its conception and subsequent reception.

The Genesis 3 narrative is palpably not a factual, historical account, but rather a myth, which conveys a particular perspective relative to a particular community at a particular time. As biblical scholar, Maretha Jacobs observes:

*'The fact that it was **their,** not **the** explanation, changes the whole matter.'* (Eve: Glimpses from her story, Scriptura 90, 2005:765-778)

I don't think my mother was operating under a curse. I don't think the pain was her fault. If anyone is to blame for the pain, blame the big baby. I caused the pain! So, shoot me, mea culpa! But in all fairness to me, the helpless baby, I didn't design the thing. I didn't ordain it to be so. And it is not my absent Dad's fault either or the absent doctors', or the incompetent nurse's. Blame Mother Nature then. The pain and all the rest of it, is...natural.

12

What was she thinking

Yes, indeed, what was Mother Nature thinking when she made it so hard and so painful? Mother Nature of course is a metaphor as Eve's Curse is a myth. The depiction Mother Nature could carry the implication of mind and design, whereas the evidence points rather to a slow, natural evolutionary process of change based on advantages and disadvantages. It is clearly an advantage to walk upright as we do, giving us the ability to see far, carry more stuff in our arms and have bigger brains, making us clever, but we don't swing very well from trees anymore and apparently our uprightness and big-brained cleverness has caused a very precarious compromise when it comes to bringing our babies into the world.

It has been called the Obstetrical Dilemma (Sherwood Washburn 1960) and it maintains that the changes to the pelvis and the development of bigger brains have caused difficult and dangerous births and abbreviated the gestation period so that our babies are born rather underdeveloped. If babies grew any bigger, they would not be able to be delivered. Bluntly stated it is the hole-and-the-head dilemma. Newer theories, like the Energetics of Gestation and Growth hypothesis (EGG) (Holly Dunsworth) emphasise the need of feeding of the baby. The baby is a little, or rather a large parasite within the mother getting all of its energy for growth from her. There comes a time when it reaches a tipping point when the mother's body cannot provide more and the baby begins to starve. This signals that it is time to abort. Yes, it seems all natural births are an abortion in some sense.

There are other interesting aspects too. Apparently, births were easier, more natural as it were, in palaeolithic times when humans were hunters and gatherers. Anthropologists point to the fact that very few infant skeletons are to be found. However, from the time when we settled and became farmers childhood mortality seemed to increase, judging by the appearance of many more tiny skeletons. One of the reasons of course is that settlement caused the spread of various forms of disease which did not occur during the nomadic lifestyle. But there is also the factor of diet. We started eating much more carbohydrates causing two further developments impacting childbirth, making it even more difficult and dangerous. First there is evidence that we became shorter and far less physically fit. This caused more changes to the bones in general and to the pelvis in particular. Secondly, we were having fatter babies due to the mother's diet, which adds more precariousness to the already tight squeeze caused by our evolution. (Cf. Colin Barras bbc.com/earth/story/201612–The real Reasons why Childbirth is so Painful and Difficult)

Whatever the exact reasons, and the scholarly situation is still dynamically developing as more research is done, it is a fact that my mother and I had a tough time that day because she was an upright walking primate and I was a big brained, Homo Sapiens baby. Although she and my father really wanted me, her body wanted me out that day. If not that day, very soon after, because there was an optimal time for me to stay otherwise, I wouldn't have got out alive. I was also beginning to cost too much in terms of her metabolism. The pains were sharp signals that the baby needed to get out, that she needed to get rid of it.

Easier said than done. We are green with envy as we look at how our mammal family cope, the relative ease and success at which they deliver their babies and the precocious state of their young. On that day in October, it would really have been easier for us if we were chimpanzees. It seems relatively easy for chimpanzees who need no assistance at all.The mother reaches down, the baby coming out facing her, takes it up to her face and starts cleaning and stimulating it. There are no chimpanzee midwives or obstetricians. Not needed at all. The chimpanzee community watch from a distance as the mother does what only the mother can and is supposed to do. If mother and I were sheep, I would have been frolicking on my four feet in minutes. But we are not. We are Homo Sapiens and that means we have developed differently from other species and also from our primate cousins

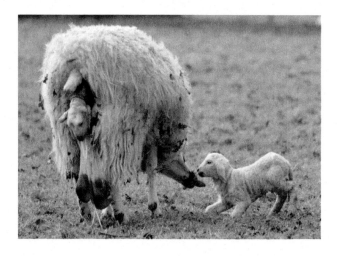

An ewe mother giving birth to twins.
Image: Karen Roe, 2012 (Creative Commons

What was Mother Nature thinking? Short answer: she wasn't.

13

Feeling it

My mother's doctor was absent, or very late, not because he was playing tennis. He could have. He had his own private tennis court. But that's not where he was. He was in theatre performing an operation, a tonsillectomy or an appendectomy, these having become popular procedures. In performing the operation, the patient would have been rendered unconscious and insensitive to pain with no memory of the procedure afterwards. My mother and I however were not in a theatre and she was fully conscious, acutely aware of every pain and remembering every second of it. What if she could also just sleep through the whole thing?

And that is exactly what Emma and Charles Darwin were thinking when they became aware of the use of chloroform. *Trichloromethane* (CHCl3) is a colourless, dense liquid, first synthesised in 1831. It was beginning to be used for all sorts of operations, but not yet for childbirth. Charles felt his beloved wife's pain deeply. After the birth of their first child in 1839 he confessed that the 'awful affair 'disturbed him very much. (Snow, 2008:80) He was a sensitive man. At medical school in Edinburgh thirteen years earlier he attended two surgical operations done without anaesthesia and he couldn't bear it. He left the operating room and soon dropped out of medical school altogether. So when they heard of the benefits of the new anaesthesia and Emma expressed the desire to have it at her next delivery, Charles did everything he could to secure it for her and to make sure it was safe, which was still a big concern at the time. He obtained chloroform through a friend and started to experiment, trying it on himself first. When Emma's delivery started unexpectedly on the 16th of August

1848, he administered it to her himself using a cloth soaked in chloroform. He kept administering it for an hour and a half, which later knowledge suggests was very dangerous, but fortunately the delivery went without problems and the baby was born painlessly. They were both very relieved and astonished at the qualities of the modern breakthrough of chloroform.

They were not the only famous couple who risked the dangers of the new substance in order to achieve a painless birth. Another celebrity of the time, Charles, Dickens, did the same as Darwin and his wife. Kate, who had a history of very difficult deliveries were as adamant and enthusiastic about using chloroform as was Emma Darwin. Dickens arranged for a skilled person from St. Bartholomew's hospital to be present at the birth and to deliver the anaesthetic. Afterwards Dickens wrote: 'The doctors were dead against it but I stood my ground, and (thank God) triumphantly. It spared her all pain. ' He said she had 'no sensation.'(Snow 2008:*82).*

About the same time, across the Atlantic in America, a similar situation occurred involving another celebrity couple concerning a different, but similar narcotic substance. Ether is a highly flammable liquid that can be vaporised into a gas. It was beginning to be used around the same time as chloroform. Fannie, the wife of the famous poet, Henry Longfellow, had heard about painless surgical and dental procedures with the use of ether and she was persuaded and also adamant that she wanted to benefit from it at the birth of their third child. They struggled to find anyone willing to agree to it. Eventually they persuaded Professor Nathan Keep, Dean of Dentistry at Harvard University to help. It was reluctantly agreed and the birth went very well. Afterwards Fannie was ecstatic about ether calling it 'the greatest blessing of this age. 'She regarded it as a 'gift of God. 'She praised God, but nevertheless felt the need to apologise for requesting and using it. She said, 'all thought me so rash and naughty in trying ether. '(Snow 2008:75)

Why was she apologising? Not mainly because the use of the drug was still new and it might be risky, but mainly because of the perception that childbirth, albeit so painful and precarious, was natural and that it should be allowed to proceed as naturally as possible. The perception was also deeply entrenched that it was ordained by God and that women should tough it out. One clergyman opined, 'Chloroform is a decoy of Satan, apparently offering itself to bless women; but in the end it will harden society and rob God of the deep earnest cries which arise in time of trouble for help. ' (Stratmann 2003:44; Snow 2008:80). Some doctors accused modern women of becoming too soft, too sophisticated, too 'posh to push. '(Epstein 2010:165). Maids, women from worker's families and women from more primitive societies were tougher and bore the burden better. Modern women's demands for help were not regarded as a sign of strength, but of weakness and the more conservative medical practitioners were, the more they were in agreement with the idea of Eve's Curse.

A big breakthrough for chloroform came in 1853 when Queen Victoria with the assistance of Prince Albert persuaded her doctors to administer it to her. By now several prominent deliveries had been performed using chloroform and the person who was most trusted in this regard was the obstetrician, John Snow. He was called to come and administer the chloroform during the birth of Prince Leopold, her eighth child, on the 7th of April. The Queen who had had a history of very difficult births were very happy about this and she testified of the tremendous relief it brought. It was not only a source of great joy, but it did much to pave the way for other mothers to be helped in the same way. It was administered again in 1857 during the birth of her last child, Princess Beatrice.

A few doors down in the Elsie Ballot hospital my mother's absent doctor was just finishing up surgery while the fortunate patient did not feel a twinge. My mother, mostly on her own, fully aware, felt it all, a century after the discovery of general anaesthesia.

14

Not Feeling it

If Charles Darwin could, he most probably would have arranged to get Emma an epidural. And Prince Albert would certainly have done the same for his beloved Queen Victoria. It would have been nice if my mother could have had one too. Epidurals are the best form of pain management in childbirth available, but it wasn't yet available during the time these people lived. As with many other forms of obstetric assistance epidurals were not first intended to help women experience less agony and discomfort during childbirth.

The first person to receive an epidural wasn't having a baby and couldn't have a baby. He was a man. Just a man, not famous, so ordinary that history has forgotten his name. And he wasn't even sick. Dr. James Leonard Corning needed a human guinea pig for research purposes. He reassured the man by telling him he had tried it on a dog and that it was fine. This was in 1885 and Corning was working in Morristown, New Jersey. Corning had studied chemistry in Stuttgart in Germany. The previous year, 1884 a German Karl Koller described the anaesthetic properties of cocaine and Corning took note of this, giving rise to his experiments. Four years later on the 16th of August 1898 another German, August Bier, performed six successful operations under spinal anaesthetic and subsequently described and published his results in the last year of the century in 1899.

In 1941 Robert Hingson and James Southworth operated on a scotsman, a merchant seaman to remove varicose veins and they inserted a needle into his lower back in an area called the cauda or the cauda equina, literally the 'horse's tail.' The spinal cord doesn't reach that far down and there is therefore no danger of damage to that vital part of the body. Instead of just giving the patient a single shot of anaesthetic, they kept the needle in, giving him several small dosages. They called this technique 'caudal continuous anaesthetic' and it was clearly very successful, but more was to come.

A few months later on the 6th of January 1942 Hingson made major medical history when his obstetrician colleague, James Edwards presented him with a pregnant patient with a rheumatic heart. It was feared that her damaged heart would not be able to withstand the rigours of natural birth and that she would also be at great risk if a Caesarean Section was performed. Hingson and Edwards decided to perform this caudal injection. The woman who was in the oh- please-Jesus-help-me-phase' of her labour, immediately became calm. Later the pain returned and Hingson was on hand to provide another dose through the already inserted needle and during this second dose the mother with the weak heart delivered her baby and both mother and child were fine. Dr Edwards made a joke by asking Hingson what he would have done if the mother didn't deliver and kept calling him throughout the night. Hingson joked that he would have had to run a small tube all the way to his bedroom from where he could simply administer another shot without having to get up and attend the patient. This joke stuck and Hingson set to work on doing just that, not running a tube all the way to his room, of course. He ran the tube up to the labouring woman's shoulder and from there subsequent dosages could easily be administered while the needle remained in her lower back area.

Dr Morris Fishbein, editor of the Journal of American Medical Association (JAMA) came to visit Dr. Hingson and wrote an article for the journal, but because he thought this technique to be of great popular interest, he also gave the story to the Readers Digest who printed it in their April Edition before it was printed in the JAMA, for which Dr. Fishbein was criticised by medical professionals. But Dr. Fishbein's sense was correct, it was a really big story, women giving birth painlessly while fully conscious and the foetus unaffected.

Epidural refers to a membrane, called the dura mater, 'strong mother' that is the outermost layer that covers the brain and the spinal cord. The space between two layers is called the epidural space. The other two are the arachnoid, meaning spider, because it looks spidery and the pia mater.

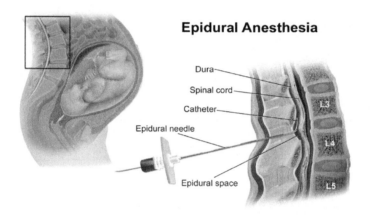

Epidural Anesthesia

PHS Medical Solutions

The dura mater is the outermost layer. And this is where a needle is placed and a catheter inserted through the needle and where small amounts of pain numbing substance is injected on a regular or continuous basis, not just a single shot.

There are differences between spinal block and an epidural. The first is a spinal anaesthetic and is useful for operations and in obstetrics for a C-section, but the epidural is a continuous pain relief where small dosages of pain relief substances can be released into the epidural space and during which a normal vaginal birth can take place with the mother fully aware but without pain.

Epidurals are now on the pain management menu for women in labour. It would have been much welcomed by people like Charles Darwin for Emma and by Prince Albert for his beloved Victoria and I think it would have been wonderful were it available to my mother and many millions of other mothers too.

15

Praise for the Poppy and the Coca!

My mother was a keen gardener. She loved plants, growing things and caring for them. She had green fingers. Plants liked her and she derived much pleasure from them. Not quite as much as she could have received had she been offered an epidural during that difficult birth when she was struggling all on her own to get me out safely. And the plant that could have been of tremendous help there is none other than the pretty little poppy, *Papaver Somniferum*. The clue is in the latin name, somniferum meaning *sleep bringing*. It is the so-called breadseed poppy. From this pretty and innocent looking plant comes opium and opioid drugs like Fentanyl and Sufentanil dripped into the epidural space from where its chemistry latches on to opioid receptors where it almost miraculously turns the pain signal settings to 'off' so that the brain doesn't know about these alarm signals.

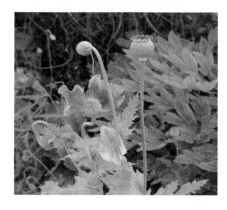

Now that is some flower power! Other well-known substances originating from this same pretty plant are morphine and the synthetically produced heroin. Everyday pain-killing substances like codeine also come from this source.

Had my plant-loving mother in her labour benefitted from the administration of an epidural, she could also have received a lot of relief from analgesic substances derived from the leaves of another plant, a black thorn bush from the *Erythroxylacae* family. The rather difficult name becomes clear, although no easier to say or write when we consider its etimology. Erythros (ερυθρός), red or ruddy in Greek and xylon (ξύλον) a Greek word for wood, or anything made of wood (xylophone and even one of the two words used for Jesus' execution stake in the New Testament!) Apart from its tricky official name it also has a more domestic name, coca plant and its leaves contain a psychoactive alcaloid called, cocaine. And yes, Coca Cola once contained a bit of this stuff in its formula which was later removed. From this plant many local anaesthetic drugs are prepared, typically ending in '-caine' like Lidocaine, mepivacaine, chlorocaine, tropocaine, encaine, holocaine, benzocaine and tetracaine. The first two, Lidocaine and Bupivacaine are frequently utilised in epidural administration. Although it is a true and a sad fact that many people suffer from addiction abusing drugs derived from these plants, in safe hands and under the right circumstances these plants and the science and technology based on it have brought enormous benefit.

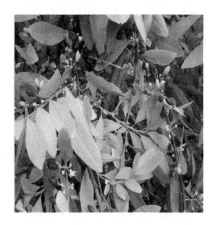

Praise then to: Papaver Somniferum and Erythrocylum Coca.

The poppy and the coca!

16

Relax, it's Natural!

Yes, indeed, childbirth is natural, just like nature intended and if you're experiencing excruciating pain, you're not doing it right. Natural in this sense also means easy and (almost) painless. Good, practical advice. Just relax about the whole thing. And who are the people offering this valuable advice? Men in white coats without wombs. There is a line in the popular sitcom, Friends, where the heavily pregnant Rachel reacts sharply to an advising man, 'No uterus, no opinion!'

The brains behind the natural birth philosophy and advice came from two men, granted they were highly skilled and trained obstetricians. They weren't just people opinionating. One was British and the other French. They were almost the same age, lived during the last half of the previous century and died within two years of each other, and although there were many points of agreement between their ideas, they were also quite different.

Dr. Ferdinand Lamaze (1891-1957) worked in Paris, but he did get quite a bit of his inspiration from Russia. His advice, developed into a system of techniques that are taught in pre-birth classes, entails the teaching of an attitude towards birth, applied in practical actions, the most important of which is to build the mother's confidence, to give her control and then of course, the famous breathing technique. Dr. Lamaze's approach was enthusiastically embraced by women, in particular the psychologist Elizabeth Bing who founded Lamaze International to promote the so-called psychoprophylactic approach to giving birth based on the French doctor's guidance.

The English doctor, Grantly Dick-Read (1890-1959), was also a well-trained doctor and obstetrician. He also thought women, modern sophisticated women to be precise, approached the whole thing wrong. They were scared and uptight, too intellectual asking too many questions and getting themselves into a knot, unlike, so-called primitive women, who just got on with it. He said, 'a tense woman closed the door to her baby.' He put his best thoughts into his book, simply entitled, Childbirth without Fear, and on a 1947 American book tour he was welcomed as a celebrity and his ideas warmly embraced. It helped too that he was an evangelical Christian. Somehow, he skipped over the so-called Curse of Eve and developed a theology of divine will. Giving birth was a blessing from God, God's intended way and it could be divine and beautiful, and with God's help and the right approach, easy and without much fuss. Feminists also loved his ideas although he was later heavily criticised by some feminists.

Evangelical believers liked his outspoken advocacy of God's way and God's presence and feminists liked that he gave women control over their bodies viewing birth not as a medical condition but as something entirely natural. It was a time when many women were marching, burning their bras in public and proudly letting their armpit hair grow and show. In the 1970's there was a celebrity-studded nationwide movement in America to de-medicalise childbirth.

There is a difference between the unassisted or free birth movement and the natural birth movement. The latter promotes birth without (unnecessary) medication and professional interventions. It is not against being assisted, but assistants could be a birth companion, a doula, and, or other helpers as well. The unassisted birth movement emphasises the natural, do-it-yourself abilities of the mother. They even go so far as connecting it with sex. Who would want to make a baby in a hospital with doctors and nurses watching and even intervening? Birth is like sex. It is love and it requires a private space and freedom, otherwise the whole thing becomes unnatural. They advocate for and practice avoidance of the involvement of professionals. They regard it as removing power and freedom from the woman. She is not sick, she is just having a baby and if her mind is in the right place, the baby and the mother will be okay.

Except, of course, that it isn't always okay and when it isn't, in the absence of expert assistance, people suffer and die. With a lot of psychological and physical preparation and in cases where no medical interventions are indicated, it can be exhilarating and feel natural and healthy. But no amount of mind over matter or healthy attitudes can save a mother and a baby when nature throws curve balls and when things go wrong.

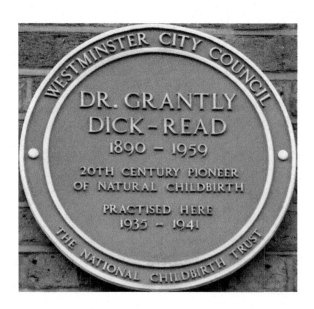

17

Breaking the silence

Idon't know how noisy or loud I was, but it wasn't quiet. Quiet is okay, it is not life threatening, as long as the baby breathes, but being totally quiet, as in still, is bad, very bad, very sad. It is sometimes even referred to as SADS, Sudden Antenatal Death Syndrome. A stillbirth is when the foetus has died, either during pregnancy or during delivery. It is not a miscarriage or a live birth. I am really glad my mother didn't suffer anyone of these two options.

It is interesting to think that the first thing a newborn does entering this world is cry, but it is quite necessary. I don't know when the practice started but doctors used to reward the new little human by holding them by the feet and slapping their bottom. It wasn't of course to punish the little fellow for being born, or to say welcome to this dreadful world or to start disciplining them right from the start. No, it was to clear the airways and encourage them to fill their lungs. I wasn't spanked because the doctor wasn't there. Maybe he should have been spanked for letting us down so badly. Today, best practice is to give the newborn a brisk rub with a towel and to apply a suction device and suck any remaining fluids out of the airways to make room for air to get right into the little lungs. Usually no stimulation is even needed because the new environment including temperature change, the lack of amniotic fluid and the exposure to air, triggers the baby's first breath. (Villines 2017:
https://www.medicalnewstoday.com/articles/318993)

It is an amazing thing if you think about it, that the baby spent nine months under water in the amniotic sac with their lungs full of amniotic fluid and the baby didn't drown! In fact, the mother did the breathing and the oxygen she breathed in reached the little one via the umbilical tube. The mother's body also got rid of the carbon-dioxide for the baby. But as soon as they are born, the baby must breathe, the lungs must be cleared of fluid and filled with air and the chord must be cut.

When I was born, I was one of about 200 born that very minute in the world. Today about 250 babies are born every minute. By the time you get to the end of this short essay there will be about 750 to a 1 000 new people in the world. Okay a lot of people also die every minute. We have not reached the point where there is a one in, one out policy, one person dies for one born and that is why the world population is growing. When I was born that day there were five billion people in the world and now there are more than seven billion. Of these births one in every forty are stillborn. In the developing world it is higher and in the developed world it is lower.

 The reasons for this SADS situation are many, the list is as long as your arm. The contributive causes are defects, diseases like malaria and diabetes, bacterial infections, smoking. Yes, what people now realise, but didn't when I was born, was that when the mother smoked, the baby also did! There are many good, predictable and preventable causes and some strange ones too, like the mother sleeping on her back after 28 weeks of pregnancy! The baby doesn't drown in the sac but could get itself really tightly entangled with the umbilical cord, which isn't usually fatal, but it could diminish the food and oxygen supply.

Stillbirth is an anti-climax, such a sad thing and a great disappointment to the mother. Pregnancy is called 'expecting' and when the baby dies before being born and is delivered without a sound or motion or any vital signs, expectation is shattered. This is why some hospitals now provide cooled 'cuddle cots' where the baby is kept for the mother to grieve and to take proper leave of the child who didn't make it safely into this world. There are even monuments and shrines where the lives of these little humans who didn't make it, are remembered. People who were born, but stillborn, who didn't scream and fill their little lungs with the air that we all live from.

I am glad I made it out safely from the little internal swimming pool where my lungs were full of liquid to the point where I let it all out, screaming or not. I am actually quite grateful I missed my first hiding and I am glad doctors and nurses have reformed themselves and stopped slapping little new arrivals, but rather giving them a brisk rubbing down with a towel.

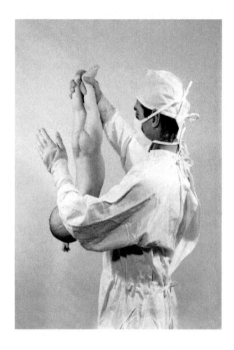

A stillbirth is not good. I am glad my mother didn't have one.

18

Picture Imperfect

My parents did not know what they were expecting. They didn't know whether I was a boy or a girl, whether I was well formed or had any potential defects. They didn't take any pre-birth pictures of me. Oh, they took loads of pictures of me after my birth, but they didn't ask for, or know about picture opportunities, Kodak moments, when I was still in the womb.

'A picture paints a thousand words' and some can kill. Taking pictures are pretty and mostly pretty harmless too. Think of the sign at picturesque and protected wildlife areas: 'Leave only footprints, take only pictures.' When photography started it looked a bit scary, the photographer hiding under a black drape and holding out a lamp that suddenly flashed a bright light like man made lightning. But everyone knew it was perfectly harmless and that it would merely produce pleasant pictures that can be kept for posterity. Say cheese!

Photography developed, pardon the pun, all sorts of pictures with a great variety of cameras. A really exciting one was a camera that could see and take pictures under the skin inside the body. A german bloke by the name of Röntgen discovered a form of light that could do just that. They were mysterious and he called them X-Rays. He took a photo of his wife's hand and only the bare bones were visible. The rays penetrated the skin and saw just the skeletal bones. He published the photo and caused a sensation in more ways than one. The minds boggled, especially the medical minds. Think of the prospects! By taking these photographs doctors would suddenly, and for the first time ever be able to look inside the body at the condition of the bones. So, if someone fell off a horse, or got punched really hard on the jaw and the doctor said, let's have a look, it was no longer a figure of speech. He, and it was still mostly males, could take an X-ray and show you the fracture. What power!

They found that they could even sneak a peek at unborn babies with these miracle rays. They could look at the cranium, the head, and all the skeletal bones of the little unborn person and it could at least give them foreknowledge whether to prepare for the C-birth. Brilliant! And so thousands of babies were subjected to these seemingly harmless photographs. But all was not well with the unborn foetuses. Gradually a horrific picture emerged. Children died from cancer and compelling scientific research pointed the accusing finger at these pictures. It became overwhelmingly clear that children exposed to these rays had a high, very high, one in two probabilities of getting Leukaemia caused by foetal, fatal, X-rays.

Appallingly and tragically many doctors didn't believe it and didn't stop. They continued shooting and killing children with these dangerous ray guns for another twenty years after the scientific study was published! Twenty years! How many children? How many children got shot in this way even before they were born, giving them a one in two chance of getting cancer in a few short years. The practice, in America only changed when insurance companies started refunding the much safer option of Sonar, ultra-sound imaging. Today, a half century or so later, with accumulated scientific data, it seems chilling that unborn babies and mothers could ever have been exposed (pardon) to these dangerous pictures. A shout out to the woman, Dr. Alice Stewart who did the scientific work and published it in 1956 in the medical journal, The Lancet. (Epstein 2011)

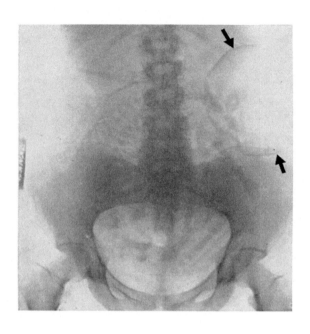

Xray image of foetus4: article by C Benson and P Doubilet, in Radiology vol 273/2014 – https://doi.org/10.1148/radiol.14140238 (Accessed 22/05/20)

I am so glad my parents took so many pictures of me as a happy baby, even some nude ones, but I am so grateful their doctor didn't point an X-ray camera at me!

19

Womb with a View

It is a privilege to look at the pictures my parents took of me as a baby. My mother made an album of the best ones, and she wrote the approximate dates under the photos: 'three months', 'nine months', and then the landmark picture at my first birthday. Lovely. These pictures show how welcome I was and how they appreciated having me. They didn't however have any pictures of me as an unborn, as a foetus. Obstetric sonography had not yet arrived in our neck of the woods.

When the 'unsinkable' Titanic hit that iceberg in 1912, it was a terrible tragedy and, in its aftermath, people began to think how great it would have been to be able to detect the presence of such a dangerous object in the dark. If 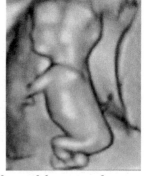 we could just see in the dark, deep waters of the ocean, it would save lives. The idea of seeing by means of sound is not alien to our world. Bats can fly safely and swiftly in the dark and dolphins can communicate and build up pictures of their environment under water and the way they do it is through sound echoing and positioning. They can echo-locate through active ultra-sound ranging. And this is what we started to do in the second world war to locate submarines.

Ultra-sound, above 20 kilohertz cannot be heard by the human ear. Dog whistles emit sounds that dogs can hear but humans cannot. So people developed these sound ranging devices which became known as SONAR: Sound Navigation and Ranging. Active sonars send out a ping and listen for the echo and in this way, it is able to build up a picture.

And so before long the technique emigrated from boats to babies. Babies, it was thought were also little submarines. It was a Scottish doctor, Ian Donald who pioneered this technique. In his article, 'Investigation of Abdominal Masses by Pulsed Ultrasound' published in the Lancet, the reputable medical journal, in 1958, he set out his ideas. Four years later a group of Americans, developed an ultrasound scanner which laid the foundation for the technology and application of ultrasound as a diagnostic method. And so a whole new world was opened, a view on the unborn baby.

In spite of fears and hesitation on the part of many obstetricians and scientists because of what happened with X-rays, the technique became popular through the decades of the sixties and seventies and by the 1980's it was becoming standard diagnostic procedure.

What is it good for? It can provide information about the condition of the pregnancy, how the baby is doing, how it is growing, the timing of the pregnancy, the size of the foetus, whether there is one gestation (baby) or more than one. On a psychological level it can help the expecting parents to bond earlier with their expected child and to prepare themselves psychologically. It can give reassurance that everything is progressing fine, and it can also help to diagnose possible defects and difficulties early. It can help with planning for the sort of delivery that can be expected. And it can reveal the sex, boy or girl.

There are cute pictures of me as a wobbly baby but there are no pictures of me as a little submarine in my mother's womb.

It wasn't yet a womb with a view.

20

A Cut Below

Growing up I had never heard of a Caesar's cut. Crew cut, yes. You'd request it at the barber's, and it relates to the style of a boy's hair. A square cut I learned about when I played cricket. A Caesar's cut is better known by the euphemistic name, Caesarean Section. It sounds softer, sensual, almost sexy. But it is definitely a cut. Not with a bat, or clippers, but with a surgical knife, a scalpel. This particular cut is done on a pregnant mother's belly to get the baby out instead of the natural way where the baby goes through the cervix and the vagina. There are two ways of doing it, longitudinally and horizontally, the latter being the more preferred method and it is rather playfully termed the bikini cut.

It is a procedure in modern obstetrics and it is now quick and quite safe, but when people first considered this method and tried it, it was in desperate circumstances. It was resorted to when the mother was either in a very bad way, unconscious, or already dead. There are stories about how people arrived at the decision. If the mother was pale, didn't move or make a sound, didn't respond to a terrible smell held under her nose and if there was no breath vapour on a mirror held in front of her mouth. That's when the priest would take charge! Of course, in those days there were no obstetricians or gynaecologists. Doctors didn't do this sort of thing. Midwives did and before there were midwives, women, friends gossips (god sibs, siblings/children of God) helped, mostly by praying, encouraging, panicking, accusing, or whatever felt right at the moment. The main reason why the priest would put down the Sword of the Spirit (The Word of God) and get a knife, was of course well intended, to save the baby, but not in the first instance to give them an opportunity at life, but in order to be able to administer eternal life-saving baptism. If the baby survived the terrible state of the mother, the crude cutting of a priest, water splashed over them and lived, that was great, of course, but if the infant, like the mother, didn't make it, the priest at least made sure they entered eternal life through baptism and blessing.

Speaking of barbers. In the early days, before modern obstetrics, barbers cut out babies for a living. They may or may not have called it the Caesar's cut, but it is doubtful. They had a wide variety of services they could perform, the barbers, associated with cutting. They had the tools. Cutting of hair was their main activity, but not as we know it, trimming and cutting hair that was thought to be too long. Men wore their hair long then. The barbers cut the hair of monks who needed a bald patch on their head. We try everything to comb over or conceal a bald patch, but back then a holy man of God needed his blessed bald patch visible. You don't want your holy, bald patch to be overgrown by hair. God forbid!

There are stories, or rather myths about the connection with Caesar maintaining that the famous emperor was born in this way, in other words that he was not born in the natural way but cut from his mother's womb. In spite of the fact that there are no good, reliable sources to corroborate this story, many people today tend to believe it.

Some attribute the procedure to Saint Caesarius of Africa, a Roman Catholic martyr. He is now regarded as the patron saint of Caesarian Sections. He is the one you'd want to pray to prior to and if possible, during the C-section. He's a good contact apparently because he is also the patron saint of flooding, drowning, lightning and earthquakes.

Modern C-sections, now perfected to a routine operation with very low risk, is a lifesaver for many and because it is elegant and easy, it has become more elective, mothers choosing the option and obstetricians offering it even in cases where there is no emergency indicated. For many mothers however this elective option is not available and in too many cases not even as an emergency option. Although some still feel strongly that 'nature's way' of vaginal birth is the best, the Caesarean has come to stay. It is undoubtably a safe, quick and relatively painless route. It does seem to be a cut above. Even though it is a cut below.

A Caesarean Section delivery
Image: HBR wiki commons 2009

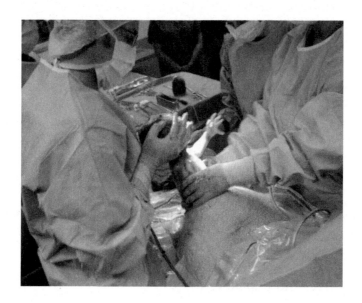

21

Forcepsed Out

Even though my birth must have been traumatic to my mother due to the disappointment of her doctor's absence and the apparent ignorance of the trainee nurse advising, 'keep it in!' the birth must have happened without any complications. She made it and I made it out. At least she was able to push me out and I was not stuck. Millions of mothers and babies have not been so lucky. Quite often the baby got stuck and this is where help was and is required. In the centuries before modern obstetrics the scene of the birth was a horror zone.

If the baby was stuck, there was a lot of poking and pushing and pulling and it got increasingly frantic. Sometimes limbs were literally pulled off. Sometimes the baby's skull was cracked, a so-called craniotomy, killing the baby to save the mother. If helpers despaired that the mother wouldn't make it, they had to make a choice, saving either one. Sometimes the baby was sacrificed to save the mother and then the treatment became really rough because the aim was no longer to deliver a live infant. If the mother was dead or dying the helpers sped up the process of getting the infant out. Sometimes an in-utero baptism was performed, sprinkling holy water into the mother. When this happened hope for a live baby was gone, giving the baby at least the hope of eternal life. After this baptism carnage ensued.

Doctors, well-meaning man-midwives employed all sorts of implements that looked a lot like medieval torture tools, knives, pokers, hooks. One such tool, the forceps has had a very long run and is still used today. It was thought that it had a very high success rate. But when it started, it was kept a secret by the inventors, the Chamberlen family in France. William Chamberlen who had inherited this secret tool from his father fled to England in 1569. The Chamberlens were Protestant Huguenots and the long persecution and war had just started in France. He passed the secret of the device and its use on to his sons and they used it among the people who could afford it. At the time people didn't travel to doctors or hospitals. The roads were terrible and there weren't any maternity wards. Local midwives assisted at births. The Chamberlens however, would visit if people had enough faith and money to employ them. They went to great lengths to keep their device a secret. They would arrive with a big box, more the size of a coffin than a toolbox, so big that two men had to carry it. They would insist that everyone leave the delivery room. People were still not really comfortable with men delivering babies. To some it bordered on adultery and there was a lot of distrust and disgust from the ranks of traditional, female midwives. They didn't trust men and their toolboxes and implements. The Chamberlens put up a sort of tent under which they worked and they blindfolded the mother. They would sneak the box in under the tent and then make all sorts of clanging noises that had nothing to do with their secret tool. They managed to keep the secret for a hundred and fifty years. In 1700 Hugh, one of the family allowed the design to go public.

The original device was discovered by sheer chance in 1813 hidden under the floorboards of a house.

Image: Chamberlen Forceps

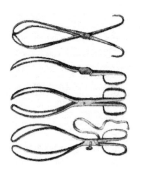

Forceps is a fairly simple device. It looks a lot like a set of tongs one would use to turn hot things on a barbeque and interestingly the two Latin words, *forum + capere* means something like hot grabber.

After baby princess Charlotte, daughter of Princess Caroline and George, Prince of Wales, the future King

George IV died in 1817 after a long and difficult labour, the obstetric assistants were criticised and accused for not using forceps to assist in her delivery. This brought a reversal of sentiments from being scared to use forceps to being more scared about not using them. It caused a great increase in the use of it.

Several other designs developed in the 19th and 20th century, from the designs by Jan Palfijn, called Palfijn's Hands, to Andre Levret's design that followed the curvature of the Pelvis and could grip higher in the birth canal, to the design published in the influential 1781 book by William Smellie, 'A Treatise on the Theory and Practice of Midwifery, to the design development by Stephen Tarnier, almost a century later in 1877, a design so successful that it was most widely used until Caesarean Sections became routine practice.

Although this 'warm' grabber fitting around the baby's head did not always work well and there were many mistakes, many injuries and casualties, if used carefully, correctly and under the right circumstances, they were a great help and one can only speculate how many mothers and babies could have been helped during the century and a half that the Chamberlens kept it secret only making their services available to the privileged people in society.

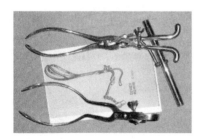

Image: Tarnier Forceps (1877)

22

Scissors, please!

It was a lovely morning in May in Sunnyside, Pretoria. The sun was up early and so were we. The sun had to be up because it was its day job and especially in Africa there is no hiding behind cloud covers. The sun puts in an honest day's work in Africa. We were also up early because my wife's contractions had started and were getting stronger and more frequent. It was time to put the pre-packed little suitcase in the yellow Volkswagen Beetle and drive the mile or two to the hospital. It was definitely time to go, but it wasn't her time yet, it was about four weeks early. Little did we know at that stage that our baby was still positioned head-up and had not yet turned. Our unborn, about to be born baby was in breech position.

Breech is a bit of a strange term. To the untrained it sounds as if the baby is in breach of some convention or rule, which in a certain sense is the case. Breech refers to the lower part of the body, and the buttocks in particular. 'Breeches' is also an old word for trousers covering the breech part of the body. About 4 out of 100 cases of full-term babies present in this upside-down position, instead of being in the downside up position, called a cephalic (head) birth. The number is a bit higher in pre-term cases, about 6%.

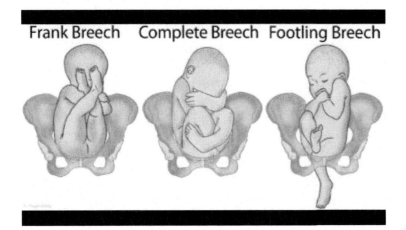

Frank Breech   Complete Breech Footling Breech

Image: Myexpertmidwife.com

There are three possible breech presentation positions: Frank Breech (sounds like a bloke's name) is when the buttocks are down, and the legs are straight up with the feet next to the foetal head. Complete Breech is when the buttocks are down, and the knees are bent with the feet near the buttocks and finally when the feet is below the buttocks it is called a Footling Breech.

Which one of these positions was going to be presented to our doctor we didn't know, but we are very grateful that he was there and exuded a wonderful calming presence, unlike the situation at my birth where the doctor exuded absence which translated into anxiety. Usually, the little fellow turns around week 36. With a full-term pregnancy there is time for the doctor to detect the position of the buttocks of the baby and perform an ECV (external cephalic version), turning the baby from the outside. With pre-term births there is no such opportunity. We were all taken by surprise and we also did not know that we were expecting a little girl.

What are some of the reasons 4% of full-termers present in this way? Various reasons are given ranging from something to do with the mother, for instance a higher incidence in mature mothers; to aspects concerning the baby, defects like hydrocephalism, or the presence of another baby, a twin, it is not uncommon in twins; or matters regarding the term, if the baby is not full term and has not yet done the turning head-down manoeuvre. In our case the main cause is likely to have been the preterm of four weeks.

I remember rather vividly the doctor announcing calmly, 'I am going to cut.' I was standing idly positioned near my wife's head. I didn't have much of a role. People were ignoring me by and large and that includes my wife. I must confess the announcement, 'I am going to cut,' sounded a bit ominous and when I started to hear the snipping sounds of the scissors a fleeting, selfish thought flashed through my mind that I hoped things down there were going to return to normal again later. But the immediate concern of course to the doctor was to deliver the buttock-down baby quickly and safely and what a great relief it was when he announced the arrival of a baby girl.

The cutting the doctor had in mind was not a C-section with a scalpel, but an episiotomy (or perineotomy) with a pair of scissors, which is the cutting of the vaginal wall to make more room. Breech births can be very dangerous because the babies' head, the largest part, comes out last and it could get stuck which could put a strain on the neck of the baby. If there is any pulling the neck and spine could be damaged leading to a condition called Erb's and Klumb's Palsy and in worst cases death. So, it is absolutely vital to create space and to deliver the baby without pulling. Pushing is the normal condition of parturition. Pulling is never a really clever idea and especially if the head comes out last and could be stuck. There are also dangers regarding compression of the umbilical cord and the oxygen supply to the baby.

After an episiotomy they sew up the cut and to my astonishment I found out reading about this that they sometimes put in an extra stitch or two which the insiders lightheartedly refer to as the 'daddy stitch', or the 'husband stitch', the purpose being to make the vagina tighter. I am sure our doctor didn't do it. I am also glad that everything healed normally, because in some cases the stitching up of the cut can cause pain during intercourse. Episiotomies are still very popular in countries like Japan and China, but it has declined precipitously in other countries of Europe (except Spain) and America. One of the reasons is probably that there is better anticipation of what sort of birth can be expected and in most cases where complications can be expected Caesarean Sections are scheduled.

23

A Mature Baby?

I was a mature baby. Now there's an oxymoron for you! I wasn't a 'premmie.' I was born at full term. Although the terms pre-mature and post-mature are still used and they refer to the state of the baby, the terms pre-term, term and post-term are preferred to refer to the stage at which birth occurred. It is a bit confusing to the uninitiated as is the dating of the pregnancy. So I will keep it simple by saying that a baby is a resident of its gracious host, the mother for 280 days or 40 weeks. Overstaying after 40 weeks is regarded as late and arriving too soon at or before week 37 is frowned upon as a bit early.

There are risks associated with babies taking a short cut to life outside. They often have a bit of liver problems, jaundice. There are possible problems with all of the organs, the kidneys, the heart, the brain—cognitive ability. There could be problems with sight and hearing and the teeth. There is a risk of cerebral palsy.

At five weeks pre-term the risk is still low and the baby has a 100% viability and chance at full health and function. Both our son and daughter were a bit early and had some problems at the start, but with good neonatal care the problems (jaundice and nasal blockage) were soon overcome. As the weeks get fewer, the baby being more early with less time in the womb, the risks at health and viability increase steadily. Our daughter's second child, a boy was born far earlier than his mother, at 31 weeks. Fortunately he was given excellent neonatal care for about six weeks and he has thankfully developed into a strong and healthy young man. At 28 weeks there is still a 90% chance, however by 25 weeks viability plunges precipitously to 50% From there on, even days are crucial. Just one week fewer, at 24 weeks, the estimated viability is only 39%. This is also more or less the earliest cut-off time allowed for an abortion: 23 weeks and 6 days (in England).

Full term consists of three terms, trimesters. During the first trimester up to twelve weeks the new life has been formed and the embryo has been implanted in the womb. The placenta is formed, and the umbilical cord provides nutrients from the mother directly to the baby. At three weeks the little one, the whole new human is really little, only 1 mm, the width of a pencil tip, or the size of a poppy seed. Three weeks later it is the size of a lentil. By 8 weeks the mother's womb is the size of a lemon. The minute little person now already has fingers and toes, eyes, a mouth and the ears are well on their way forming. From week 12 onward, professionals change the title and start calling it a foetus. It has made it through the embryo phase, and it is now a fully formed foetus! The little heart has started beating. The foetus is the size of a small apple, and it already has a beating heart!

And into the second exciting trimester the little fellow, boy or girl goes. By the way at fertilisation 23 chromosomes from the father and 23 from the mother unite. A human is made up of 46 of these tiny, really tiny, little stringy things. But do not underestimate their potency. Each one contains 2 000 genes, and each gene contains vital information for the building of the unique human being. The baby now starts to move, flex its arms and legs for exercise while all the other organs continue to develop at pace. Around 17 weeks brain function starts up. The baby practices mock breathing although the lungs are still full of the amniotic fluid. The baby can swallow, and the kidneys and digestive system starts to work in a preparatory way with bits of pee and poo excreted (sorry mum!). From week 27 we are reaching the home stretch. Baby will start opening his or her eyes and cute little eyelashes form. It might also have a full head of hair. They will gain a lot more in size and weight, now about 10 inches long and 1 kilogram, like a bar of butter! From week 31 there is a rapid weight gain and putting on of fat in order to prepare it for the big climate change that is going to happen soon. The central nervous system is up and running, directing rhythmic breathing movements and controlling autonomous body temperature. At 33 weeks the pupils of the eyes can change in response to stimuli. In another three weeks the baby will decide, naturally that it is a good idea to go for a dive, turning itself head down, the head moving into the pelvic cavity between the mother's hips. Around 38 weeks the baby's head and belly are of equal

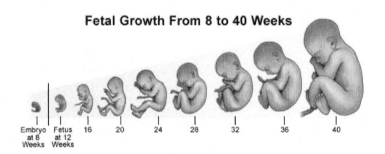

Fetal Growth From 8 to 40 Weeks

Embryo at 8 Weeks   Fetus at 12 Weeks   16   20   24   28   32   36   40

size and the weight might be up to three kilograms. Within the next days and hours the signs and signals, the contractions and downward movement will start and a brand new, unique human individual will be added to the world.

Even though I was a mature baby at the time of my birth, I was a typical human which means I was utterly immature, infantile and helpless at birth and for a very long time thereafter.

Image: Brgfx freepik.com

24

In search of my I

That day when the doctor was absent and mother struggled alone in her labour, I was there. He and I were both expected, but he was absent while I was definitely present. My mother knew I was there. She had known for a long time. Everyone knew. They could see me. I was the bump. Although I was undeniably there, 'on the way' and even though I was clearly visibly there at the moment of my birth when the doctor wasn't, I didn't know it. Even though I was a mature baby (full term, that is), it took a very long time for me to know anything.

The first things I know I knew was when I was about four years old. I must be careful with this because there are many things I know of and can remember, but not because I knew them firsthand. Many things I know of my early years are from stories I were told about myself. I knew later what I didn't know earlier.

Knowing is a slippery term. Does a baby know they are uncomfortable, cold, wet hungry or has cramps? Quite clearly yes, based on the insistent and incessant crying and on the contentment when the particular need they were screaming about is met. Even though the baby has not yet acquired word power and has no frame of reference in their brain, they can 'know' certain things and even find a primitive way of communicating them. Parents have to use their brain power to 'read' what the infant is trying to 'say'. It is clear that before the acquisition of language 'knowing' and 'saying' should best be furnished with inverted commas. It is a knowing but not as we know it.

So when did I start? When was I there? Clearly everything I have, anatomically and physically was already formed and functioning long before I was born. I had a brain when I was but a bump in a belly. I had a beating heart when I was living in an amniotic sac. So let's go back right to the start when the little champion sperm who would win the day was still zig-zagging frenetically in its quest to find the egg. Clearly that was not I. That was a loaded, coded, moving messenger stick full of data from my dad.

And when that cute little oocyte started its journey along the fallopian way it wasn't my mother, but it contained the other half of my rudimentary genetic information. I was not there yet. But when these two met it was magic. One moment there were two and then there was one. And that one was I.

I, just me, 'not my mama, not papa but it's me, oh Lord,' as the old spiritual song goes.

It could never be anyone else already when I was two cells, four cells, a ball of twelve cells, even before that ball found its home in the womb where its wellbeing would be secured for all of the time it needed to develop eyes, ears, organs, hands, toes, feet and all of the features of a physical body. That physical body was always and only going to become me. Actually, it was me, embryonic I. It is the same brain that was there in the womb then that enables me to work now. It had just developed. When I was in the womb I just lacked the word power.

The clue it seems is conception, a unique configuration of cells. Given time and temperate conditions, cognition commences, developing into consciousness and eventually communication. I am, therefore, I think.

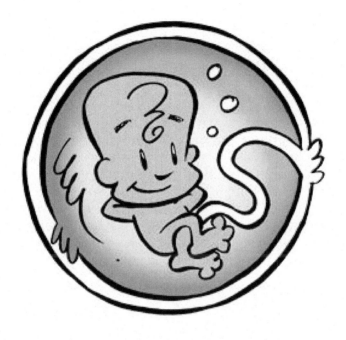

{Image:Umbert the Unborn by Gary Cangemi

I think I have found my I

25

Well Connected

In a previous chapter above I celebrated the fact of my uniqueness, the astounding thought that there is no-one quite like me. In this chapter I want to celebrate the opposite idea, that I have things in common with other people and that this mutuality makes me not-so unique after all. Although I am one of a kind, I am intimately related to the kind that I am one of. What I have every human being also has and had. I am related to that individual who lived on the African savannah fifty thousand years ago. He, like me, had two legs, two arms, a head with two eyes, two ears, a nose, a nervous system that could warn him of danger. The same nervous system that conveys messages to my brain as I negotiate the intricacies of reading, writing and riding a motorcycle in traffic or in the rain, worked exactly the same for him as he set out to track prey for food and listen for possible predators who might regard him as food. Humans are estimated to be more than 99% genetically similar. We all share a shed load of stuff.

And it doesn't stop there. We are quite closely related to other primates. Their genome and ours are very similar to a high percentage, more than 98 % in the case of chimpanzees and even the bit more distant gorillas. And it is not difficult to see. Although there are clear and obvious differences between me and a gorilla, it is also blatantly obvious that we share a lot. Look at the body plan, head, eyes, ears, nose, mouth, the internal organs with the same functions, a long list of similarities. And if we fast forward, or rather rewind all the way along the branch of mammals, we can see the same shared sameness even in mice and rats. Because they are so similar to us, they have been used for medical trials ultimately aimed to benefit humans. In spite of our clear and obvious differences we are related in a multitude of ways.

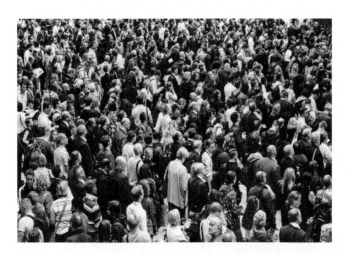 Biologist Richard Dawkins uses the metaphor of a river of genes flowing through individual bodies through time. And this river emanates from a metaphorical Eden where the first life forms started. All life ultimately has a single common ancestor. That means I am genetically related to all multi-celled and single-celled forms of life. I am related to bacteria and the intimacy between us is graphically demonstrated by the fact that even though my body contains something in the order of 30 trillion cells, it hosts even more single-celled organisms that call my body home! Relatedness, sharedness on a microbial level.

My shared relatedness does not stop when we leave the realm of genes. On an atomic level, I share stuff with rocks, and rivers, the air, the sky, space and the stars. My body is made up of the chemical elements produced in space, by the so-called Big Bang when matter was made. Hydrogen, the lightest and most abundant element is essential to the making and functioning of my body, but also of so much else in the physical world. Carbon, the 6th heaviest element, created in the cauldrons of stars, make up a very high percentage of the bodies of everything, including mine. Life is carbon based and this essential element was once produced in the factory that is a star. My body also shares atomic elements, joined as molecules, like water, essential to life, but again, had its genesis in the life and death of stars. The heavier elements all came from super-massive stars and supernova explosions at the end of their lives. It has been said, and it is literally true, that we are made of star stuff. Without the life and death of stars I wouldn't be alive.

I am bowled over, baffled, in awe of how widely and deeply I am related on the basis of stuff shared with almost everything else from as small as atoms to as big as the biggest stars and galaxies thousands of light years away. As the song says, 'we are family' and it applies to absolutely everything.

I am unique. And Not. And so are you.

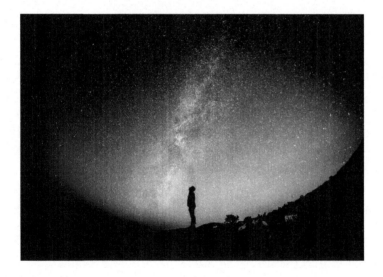

Photo credits Crowd: Rob Curren, <u>unsplash.com</u>

Stars: Greg Rakozy, <u>unsplash.com</u>

Sources and Further Reading

Epstein, R. H. 2010, *Get Me Out. A History of Childbirth from the Garden of Eden to the Sperm Bank.* London, New York: W. W. Norton & Company.

Kitzinger, S. 2003, *The New Pregnancy & Childbirth. Choices and Challenges.* London: Dorling Kindersley Ltd.

Snow, S. J. 2008, *Blessed Days of Anaesthesia. How Anaesthetics Changed the World.* Oxford: Oxford University Press.

Stone, A. 2019, *Being Born. Birth and Philosophy.* Oxford: Oxford University Press

Printed in Great Britain
by Amazon

16385594R10051